Getting Started in Non-Sterile Compounding Video Training Program

WORKBOOK

American Society of Health-System Pharmacists®
Bethesda, Maryland

Any correspondence regarding this publication should be sent to the publisher, American Society of Health-System Pharmacists, 7272 Wisconsin Avenue, Bethesda, MD 20814, attention: Special Publishing.

Director, Special Publishing: Jack Bruggeman
Acquisitions Editor and Video Producer: Hal Pollard
Senior Editorial Project Manager and Script Editor: Dana Battaglia
Script and Workbook Writing Services: Sellers Communications
Film Direction: Frank Lama, ICS Learning Group
Video Production: Odyssey
Production: Johnna Hershey, David Wade
Package Design: Armen Kojoyian

ISBN: 978-1-58528-189-3

Program Consultants and Subject Matter Experts

Karen Davis, CPhT, is the Pharmacy Technology Director and an instructor at the Southeastern Technical College in Vidalia, Georgia. She has practiced as a pharmacy technician for over 27 years in both retail and hospital settings.

Jason Sparks, AAS, BA, CPhT, PhTR, is an Assistant Professor and Clinical Coordinator at Austin Community College in Austin, Texas. He is president-elect of the Pharmacy Technician Educators Council.

Acknowledgment

ASHP would like to acknowledge the assistance of the University of Maryland School of Pharmacy, especially Dr. Richard Dalby.

Table of Contents

Program Consultants and Subject Matter Experts iii

Introduction vii

Section 1: Dosage Forms

Exercise A Word Search: Compounding Dosage Forms 2
Exercise B Crossword Puzzle: Do You Know Your Dosage Forms? 3
Exercise C Short Answer Quiz 4
Exercise D Multiple Choice Questions 5
Exercise E Fill in the Blank Exercises 6
Exercise F Match Dosages and Preparations 7

Section 2: Equipment

Exercise A Word Search: Compounding Equipment 10
Exercise B Crossword Puzzle: Do You Know Your Compounding Equipment? 11
Exercise C Short Answer Quiz 12
Exercise D Multiple Choice Questions 13
Exercise E Fill in the Blank Exercises 14
Exercise F Match the Equipment with Its Function 15

Section 3: Packaging

Exercise A Word Search: Packaging 18
Exercise B Crossword Puzzle: Do You Know Your Packaging? 19
Exercise C Short Answer Quiz 20
Exercise D Multiple Choice Questions 21
Exercise E Fill in the Blank Exercises 22
Exercise F Match Dosage Forms with the Correct Packaging 23

Section 4: Techniques

Exercise A Word Search: Compounding Technique 26
Exercise B Crossword Puzzle: Do you Know Your Compounding Techniques and Terminology? 27
Exercise C Short Answer Quiz 28
Exercise D Multiple Choice Questions 29
Exercise E Fill in the Blank Exercises 30
Exercise F Match the Dosage Form with the Correct Technique or Preparation 31

Section 5: Compounding Exercises

Pharmacy Compounding Log 34
300,000 Unit Nystatin Hard Lozenges 35
Zinc Oxide Paste 36
88% Isopropyl Alcohol 37
Apple Pie Capsules 38
Metronidazole 500 mg/5 mL Oral Suspension 39
Magic Mouthwash (4:2:1) 40

Answer Key 41
Glossary 47
Index 51

Introduction

Welcome to the *Getting Started in Non-Sterile Compounding Video Training Program* accompanying workbook! This workbook tests your knowledge of non-sterile compounding dosage forms, terminology, equipment, and techniques. The exercises within this workbook are designed to complement the video/DVD to educate you on the basics of compounding non-sterile preparations.

How to Use This Program

This training program allows you to work at your own pace. The video/DVD and workbook complete the training program. The workbook is designed to support the video/DVD content by using exercises developed to reinforce key concepts and skills presented in the video/DVD as well as to strengthen your vocabulary.

You do not have to complete the exercises while viewing the video/DVD, but rather familiarize yourself with the content, then return, at a later time, to complete each exercise. The workbook also contains a glossary of terms you should know. **Note:** This program is not intended to replace or demonstrate best "hands-on" practices but rather provide an overview of the non-sterile compounding and a foundation for best practices.

You should work through the entire program first before reviewing any sections out of sequence.

You are now invited to begin. Good luck, and enjoy the program!

SECTION 1

Dosage Forms

Learning Objectives

After watching the video/DVD, you should be able to

1. Recognize and define terminology related to compounded dosage forms.
2. Describe the major differences between dosage forms.
3. Identify the reasons why non-sterile compounding occurs.
4. Discuss the reasons why one dosage form would be used instead of another.
5. Match a commercially available product with its appropriate dosage form.
6. Discuss special compounding techniques used with each dosage form.

Exercise A – Word Search: Compounding Dosage Forms

Find the following words and circle them.

AROMATICSOLUTIONS
CAPSULES
CREAMS
ELIXIRS
EMULSIONS
EXTRACTS
LOTIONS
LOZENGES
OINTMENTS
PASTES
POWDERS
SUPPOSITORIES
SUSPENSIONS
SYRUPS
TINCTURES

P	K	S	E	R	U	T	C	N	I	T	Y	L	S	X	S	T	D
T	P	O	W	D	E	R	S	L	B	S	B	M	U	Y	N	P	E
N	N	S	M	R	W	M	Q	J	Y	K	R	C	S	V	O	K	M
L	D	K	U	Z	T	T	M	R	K	Y	F	E	P	B	I	P	U
R	N	Q	H	P	F	Y	U	C	F	J	X	C	E	P	T	S	L
N	Z	G	H	H	P	P	E	Z	L	T	T	V	N	H	U	T	S
X	W	N	L	N	S	O	W	L	R	L	C	F	S	B	L	N	I
V	H	K	M	L	J	W	S	A	I	M	V	E	I	L	O	E	O
C	R	E	A	M	S	Z	C	I	N	X	L	D	O	K	S	M	N
D	B	J	J	C	S	T	N	H	T	U	I	X	N	T	C	T	S
G	V	Z	Z	D	S	E	R	R	S	O	X	R	S	G	I	N	R
T	B	P	Q	N	R	C	G	P	P	H	R	E	S	K	T	I	C
T	Q	X	N	Z	R	T	A	N	L	K	T	I	Y	T	A	O	K
Z	V	T	J	V	C	C	Z	M	E	S	L	K	E	T	M	R	N
K	F	K	Y	L	M	L	Q	F	A	Z	P	B	M	S	O	X	G
B	L	P	D	D	T	H	B	P	M	R	O	N	M	F	R	W	R
J	S	N	O	I	T	O	L	M	L	C	M	L	X	T	A	N	J

Answers on page 41.

Exercise B – Crossword Puzzle: Do You Know Your Dosage Forms?

Use the clues given to fill in the puzzle.

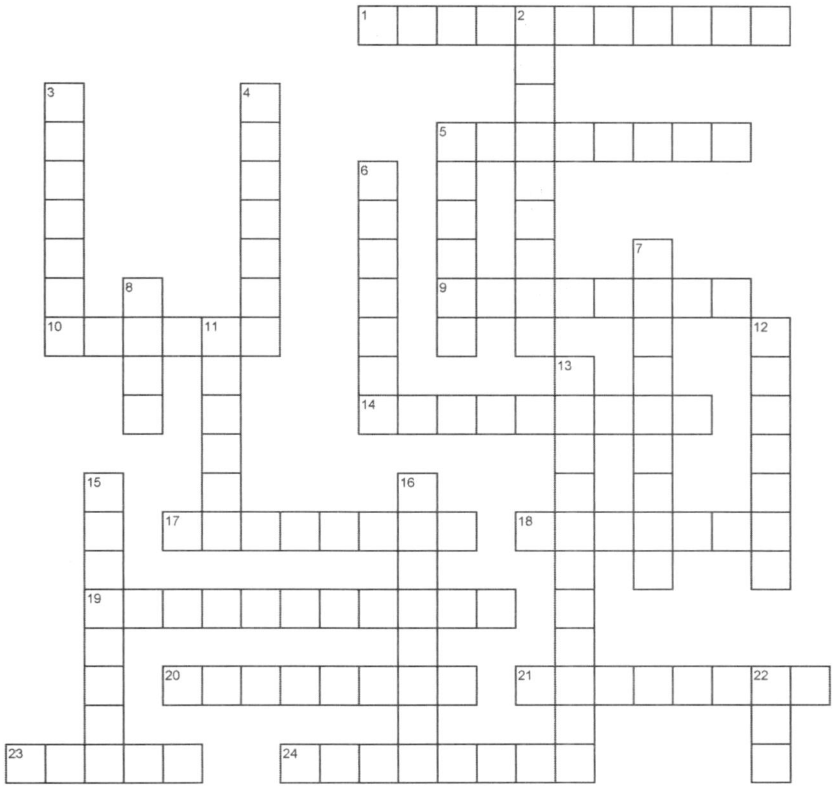

ACROSS

1 _______ must be shaken prior to administration because of non-dissolved particles.
5 Dosage form known as a medication stick.
9 Triple antibiotic is an example.
10 ______ are thick solutions with high sugar content.
14 Oral solution not mentioned previously in this exercise.
17 _______ solutions have a strong smell.
18 Petroleium jelly is used to prepare a ______ preparation.
19 Common base for suppositories.
20 May be contained in capsules.
21 Aqueous, alcoholic, and hydroalcoholic refer to the base of a ________.
23 Leaves a greasy feeling on skin.
24 A suppository can be given _______.

DOWN

2 Lotions and creams are _______.
3 _______ are typically clear, sweet, and flavored solutions.
4 ______ were the only dosage forms not discussed in the video.
5 Apply smoothly to skin.
6 A type of solution from plant or animal sources.
7 ________ dilution.
8 Take by mouth.
11 Sifting and tumbling are used to prepare this dosage form.
12 Made of vegetable gelatin.
13 Melting and chilling are used in preparing this dosage form.
15 Lozenges are also known as _______.
16 Water in oil emulsion.
22 Water in oil emulsions contain more of this than water.

Answers on page 41.

Exercise C – Short Answer Quiz

The video/DVD listed six reasons for non-sterile compounding. List four of them here.

1. ______________________________

____

2. ______________________________

____

3. ______________________________

____

4. ______________________________

____

Answers on page 41.

Exercise D – Multiple Choice Questions

Select the best answer to each of the following questions.

1. **The following routes require non-sterile compounding, except**
   A. Vaginal.
   B. Ophthalmic.
   C. Rectal.
   D. Oral.

2. **Compounding has been likened to**
   A. Baking a cake.
   B. Washing a car.
   C. Riding a bike.
   D. Walking a dog.

3. **If a medication is not prepared according to the recipe, the following could happen:**
   A. Patient could get too much medication.
   B. Patient could die.
   C. Patient could get too little medication.
   D. All of the above.

4. **Reasons to compound include all of the following, except**
   A. Customized rate of delivery.
   B. Customized rate of onset.
   C. Dosage form not available.
   D. Dosage form too expensive.

5. **All of the following are patient populations that could benefit from non-sterile compounding, except**
   A. Patients who cannot swallow.
   B. Patients who need smaller doses.
   C. Patients who need intravenous medications.
   D. Patients who cannot tolerate certain tastes.

6. **Phenobarbital elixir is an example of which of the following bases?**
   A. Hydroalcoholic.
   B. Alcoholic.
   C. Water.
   D. Aqueous.

7. **The primary tools used in preparing creams, ointments, and pastes are**
   A. Beaker and test tube.
   B. Slab and spatula.
   C. Pipette and flask.
   D. Mortar and pestle.

8. **Oral capsules may contain all of the following, except**
   A. Granules.
   B. Cream.
   C. Powder.
   D. Liquid.

9. **The outer shell of a capsule is made of gelatin so that it will**
   A. Dissolve easily.
   B. Be absorbed easily.
   C. Be distributed easily.
   D. All of the above.

10. **Suppositories may be inserted into the**
    A. Nasal passage.
    B. Urethra.
    C. Ear canal.
    D. All of the above.

11. **Lozenges are for patients who**
    A. Cannot take medications.
    B. Cannot chew.
    C. Cannot swallow.
    D. Cannot taste.

12. **Powders are prepared by which of the following methods?**
    A. Dilution.
    B. Grinding.
    C. Mixing.
    D. Crushing.

13. **Chilling suppositories ensures that the active ingredient**
    A. Stays active in the base.
    B. Remains suspended in the base.
    C. Dissolves in the base.
    D. Settles in the base.

14. **Oil-in-water preparations include the following, except**
    A. Creams.
    B. Lotions.
    C. Ointments.
    D. Benzoyl peroxide.

15. **Syrups contain a large amount of the following, except**
    A. Sugar.
    B. Sweetener.
    C. Sorbitol.
    D. Water.

Answers on page 41.

Exercise E – Fill in the Blank Exercises

1. The best base to use in a solution is determined by the ________________.
2. Powders must be uniform in ____________ and ____________ in order to be maximally utilized.
3. Compounding suppositories starts with _____________ the base and then adding the _________________.
4. Suppositories and suspensions contain __________________ particles.
5. Extracts and _____________ can come from plant sources.
6. Elixirs usually have a _______________ base.
7. Thickening agents are added to _______________.
8. Vaseline™, Aquaphor™, and Eucerin™ may be used as bases for ________, ________, ________________, and ________________.
9. Ointments and pastes are _________________ emulsions.
10. Suspensions are _________________-based solutions.
11. Cough syrups are typically _________________-based solutions.
12. Suspensions are ________________ prior to administration.
13. Tinctures may have a ________________ or __________________ base.
14. Geometric dilution is a compounding ___________________.
15. The drug dosage form is also known as the ___________________________ (three words).

Answers on page 41.

Exercise F – Match Dosages and Preparations

Match the preparation on the left with the dosage form on the right.

_____ 1. Calamine	A. Ointment
_____ 2. Hydrocortisone	B. Paste
_____ 3. Glycerin	C. Lotion
_____ 4. Triple antibiotic	D. Cream
_____ 5. Zinc oxide	E. Suppositories

Answers on page 42.

SECTION 2

Equipment

Learning Objectives

After watching the video/DVD, you should be able to

1. Recognize and define terminology related to compounding equipment.
2. Describe the major differences between containers used for liquid measurements.
3. Identify the pros and cons of balances used in compounding.
4. Discuss the reasons why one mortar and pestle would be used over another.
5. Match a piece of equipment with its appropriate function.
6. Discuss special compounding techniques used with compounding equipment.

Exercise A – Word Search: Compounding Equipment

Find the following words and circle them.

ALUMINUM
BEAKERS
BULBSYRINGE
CALIBRATIONMARKS
DIGITALBALANCE
FORCEPS
GELATINCAPSULES
GRADUATEDCYLINDERS
MORTARANDPESTLE
OINTMENTSLAB
PARCHMENTPAPER
PIPETTES
PURIFIEDWATER
RUBBERSPATULA
STAINLESSSTEELSPATULA
SUPPOSITORYMOLD
SYRINGES
TWOPANBALANCE
VOLUMETRICFLASKS
WEIGHINGBOATS

G	R	A	D	U	A	T	E	D	C	Y	L	I	N	D	E	R	S	Z	V	R
J	V	D	D	N	Q	H	P	D	T	G	K	W	F	N	K	Y	M	J	N	D
A	L	U	T	A	P	S	L	E	E	T	S	S	S	E	L	N	I	A	T	S
B	K	G	S	U	P	P	O	S	I	T	O	R	Y	M	O	L	D	D	T	Z
T	T	B	X	G	V	N	R	C	D	Y	R	L	L	L	C	R	V	I	T	C
P	Z	S	E	L	U	S	P	A	C	N	I	T	A	L	E	G	R	G	M	R
H	I	T	W	Z	T	V	T	L	M	P	V	T	T	R	W	E	B	I	B	V
E	H	P	H	X	W	L	B	L	T	J	Z	M	U	J	P	P	S	T	N	L
P	L	H	E	H	M	G	L	H	K	N	W	B	R	A	H	G	K	A	D	P
C	M	T	X	T	B	L	B	R	L	C	B	F	P	W	K	R	S	L	R	U
N	A	B	S	D	T	X	N	Q	J	E	X	T	T	N	F	M	A	B	L	R
L	M	L	J	E	G	E	L	C	R	W	N	L	X	R	F	N	L	A	D	I
W	R	T	I	R	P	L	S	S	V	E	P	H	J	R	R	L	F	L	V	F
N	Q	G	L	B	H	D	P	S	M	C	H	N	K	Y	P	P	C	A	T	I
K	W	V	Q	Y	R	A	N	H	E	B	U	L	B	S	Y	R	I	N	G	E
B	Z	M	L	N	T	A	C	A	T	G	D	K	T	J	L	R	R	C	Y	D
A	F	Y	Z	U	K	R	T	K	R	R	N	A	P	R	M	M	T	E	G	W
L	J	N	L	P	A	D	K	I	N	A	O	I	J	K	Q	M	E	R	N	A
S	Z	A	T	P	G	Y	F	R	O	B	T	T	R	G	X	U	M	L	T	T
T	P	M	R	G	V	O	T	Y	G	N	S	R	H	Y	Y	N	U	Z	C	E
N	K	G	M	Y	R	G	M	N	Q	R	M	L	O	K	S	I	L	R	H	R
E	T	D	G	C	K	D	I	F	E	T	H	A	K	M	F	M	O	B	H	T
M	G	V	E	T	X	H	N	K	L	F	R	W	R	G	P	U	V	Z	N	W
T	V	P	K	Q	G	R	A	J	N	R	P	D	M	K	P	L	B	N	T	N
N	S	K	R	I	G	E	D	M	R	K	L	C	X	K	S	A	M	M	N	M
I	B	X	E	T	B	Q	L	B	P	K	J	L	L	Q	G	H	W	R	L	Z
O	Y	W	L	T	E	C	N	A	L	A	B	N	A	P	O	W	T	N	P	M

Answers on page 42.

Exercise B – Crossword Puzzle: Do You Know Your Compounding Equipment?

Use the clues given to fill in the puzzle.

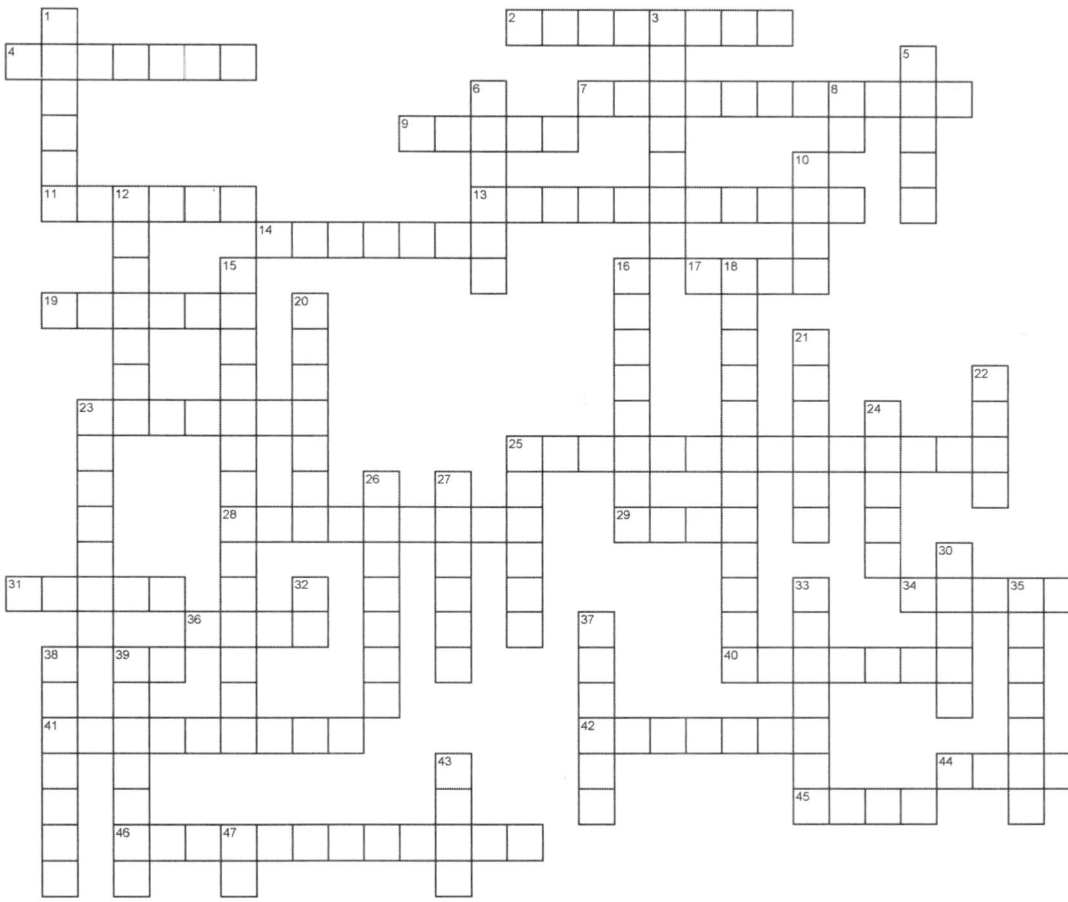

ACROSS

2 Reading the ________.
4 Used to pick up small weights.
7 Type of mixing technique.
9 Suppository _______.
11 Hard ______ spatula.
13 Type of mixing technique.
14 Used to pick up small weights.
17 A gelatin shell part.
19 Two pan balance.
23 Metric or apothecary.
25 Protects counters from damage and mess.
28 Surface of ointment slab is ________.
29 Other type of gelatin shell.
31 Purified _____ is important in compounding.
34 Small mouth and narrow neck.
36 One type of gelatin shell.
39 Abbreviation for "to deliver".
40 Used to measure liquid ingredients.
41 Surface of ointment slab is _________.
42 Another name for scale.
44 Type of syringe used with pipettes.
45 Other type of gelatin shell.
46 Thick piece of glass used in spatulation.

DOWN

1 Equipment most often associated with pharmacy practice. (first word)
3 Double-sided blade used for mixing.
5 Suppository _______.
6 Two pan balance.
8 Abbreviation for "to contain".
10 A gelatin shell part.
12 Another name for scale.
15 Protects counters from damage and mess.
16 Reading the _________.
18 Thick piece of glass used in spatulation.
20 Surface _______.
21 Equipment most often associated with pharmacy practice. (second word)
22 One type of gelatin shell.
23 Metric or apothecary.
24 Purified ______ is important in compounding.
25 Equipment most often associated with pharmacy practice (second word).
26 Shape of the meniscus.
27 Equipment most often associated with pharmacy practice (first word).
30 Small mouth and narrow neck.
32 Abbreviation for "to deliver".
33 Used to measure liquid ingredients.
35 Double-sided blade used for mixing.
37 Hard _______ spatula.
38 Shape of the meniscus.
39 Surface _______.
43 Type of syringe used with pipettes.
47 Abbreviation for "to contain."

Answers on page 42.

Exercise C – Short Answer Quiz

The video/DVD discussed compounding suppositories and the various molds used in preparing them. Please provide the reason molds are necessary and the three most common types of molds used.

Answers on page 42.

Exercise D – Multiple Choice Questions

Select the best answer to each of the following questions.

1. Single pipettes are designed to deliver
   A. Single fixed volumes and no partial amounts.
   B. Single fixed volumes and partial amounts.
   C. Multiple fixed volumes and no partial amounts.
   D. Multiple fixed volumes and partial amounts.

2. Syringes may be used for all of the following except
   A. Injecting.
   B. Withdrawing.
   C. Irrigating.
   D. Puncturing.

3. Which of the following is a type of syringe tip?
   A. Slide tip.
   B. Luer lock tip.
   C. Rectal tip.
   D. Screw tip.

4. Suppository molds may be made of the following except
   A. Plastic.
   B. Aluminum.
   C. Lead.
   D. All of the above.

5. Spatulas perform which of the following functions?
   A. Counting.
   B. Transferring.
   C. Mixing.
   D. All of the above.

6. Stainless steel spatulas are
   A. Somewhat flexible.
   B. Resistant to bending.
   C. Not helpful in spatulation.
   D. Not helpful in mixing.

7. Ointment slabs are usually made of
   A. Thick glass.
   B. Thick plastic.
   C. Thick plexi-glass.
   D. All of the above.

8. Mortars and pestles may be made of the following:
   A. Ceramic.
   B. Glass.
   C. Wood.
   D. All of the above.

9. Using a scale or balance properly ensures which of the following?
   A. Correct dosage.
   B. Correct mixing.
   C. Correct ingredient.
   D. All of the above.

10. Two-pan balance is used to weigh
    A. Small amounts.
    B. Medium amounts.
    C. Large amounts.
    D. Huge amounts.

11. Standardized weights are used to weigh
    A. Powders
    B. Granules.
    C. Ointments.
    D. All of the above.

12. Which of the following most accurately describes a beaker?
    A. Small-mouthed.
    B. Durable.
    C. Hold medium amounts.
    D. No spout.

13. Which of the following most accurately describes a volumetric flask?
    A. Large-mouthed.
    B. Wide neck.
    C. Wide base.
    D. No spout.

14. Which of the following most accurately describes a graduated cylinder?
    A. Transfers liquids only.
    B. Measures liquids only.
    C. Measures and transfers liquids only.
    D. Does not measure or transfer liquids.

15. Which of the following most accurately describes a pipette?
    A. Delivers amounts greater than 25 milliliters.
    B. Delivers amounts 25 milliliters or less.
    C. Delivers amounts less than 25 milliliters.
    D. None of the above.

Answers on page 42.

Exercise E – Fill in the Blank Exercises

1. _______________ are used to protect balances from contamination.
2. A _______________ is much easier to use and more accurate than the Class A balance.
3. _______________ may be cylindrical or conical, plastic or glass.
4. Cylindrical graduated cylinders are more accurate than ____________ graduated cylinders.
5. Plastic ____________ syringes are used most often when compounding non-sterile preparations.
6. Slip tips have large openings that assist in drawing up ____________ fluids.
7. The ____________ method is used to filled gelatin capsules with powder.
8. Weighing boats are made of _______________.
9. Weighing papers are used to measure and ___________ smaller quantities.
10. Parchment paper is used in place of an _______________.
11. Mortar is a ____________, and the pestle is the _____________.
12. A _______________ is used when measuring with a digital balance to protect the ingredient.
13. Calibrated pipettes can deliver ____________ and ____________ amounts.
14. Syringes may be used to mix and ____________ medications.
15. Syringes are composed of a ____________ and ____________.

Answers on page 42.

Exercise F – Match the Equipment with Its Function

Match the piece of equipment on the left with its function on the right.

_____ 1.	Mortar	A.	Transfer ingredients from balance
_____ 2.	Beaker	B.	Pounder/grinder
_____ 3.	Pipette	C.	Can be substituted for an ointment slab
_____ 4.	Syringe	D.	Mixing liquid or semi-solid dosage forms
_____ 5.	Pestle	E.	Used to weigh ingredients
_____ 6.	Spatula	F.	Bowl for mixing
_____ 7.	Balance	G.	Mixing and giving medication
_____ 8.	Ointment slab	H.	Measure or transfer large volumes of liquid
_____ 9.	Parchment paper	I.	Measure or transfer small volumes of liquid
_____10.	Weighing paper	J.	Nonporous surface used for mixing ointment

Answers on page 42 and 43.

SECTION 3

Packaging

Learning Objectives

After watching the video/DVD, you should be able to

1. Recognize and define terminology related to preparation packaging.
2. Describe the necessary documentation elements for packages.
3. Identify the pros and cons of packages used in compounding.
4. Discuss why the appropriate package is important.
5. Match a compounded dosage form with its appropriate package.
6. Discuss other elements to consider as part of the packaging process.

Exercise A – Word Search: Packaging

Find the following words and circle them.

ALUMINUMWRAPS
DATING
DOCUMENTATION
GLASSBOTTLES
LABELING
OINTMENTJARS
OINTMENTTUBES
PACKAGING
PLASTICBOTTLES
STORING

K	H	N	K	X	D	F	F	P	J	X	O	S	C	D
N	W	L	X	T	C	K	A	V	B	W	I	P	S	X
Y	Q	P	A	R	Z	C	D	L	R	R	N	A	E	Z
P	R	G	B	B	K	T	T	H	D	M	T	R	B	K
R	W	C	N	A	E	X	G	G	M	N	M	W	U	L
M	T	J	G	I	X	L	N	V	N	T	E	M	T	L
T	L	I	K	R	R	I	I	W	K	R	N	U	T	G
T	N	Q	H	L	T	O	W	N	L	W	T	N	N	L
G	R	X	N	A	Q	M	T	Q	G	T	J	I	E	V
X	J	T	D	T	M	K	L	S	N	T	A	M	M	X
L	D	Y	P	M	T	W	Q	Y	H	G	R	U	T	J
G	L	A	S	S	B	O	T	T	L	E	S	L	N	K
N	D	P	R	N	C	C	X	W	G	C	Z	A	I	L
L	N	N	O	I	T	A	T	N	E	M	U	C	O	D
S	E	L	T	T	O	B	C	I	T	S	A	L	P	N

Answers on page 43.

Exercise B – Crossword Puzzle: Do You Know Your Packaging?

Use the clues given to fill in the puzzle.

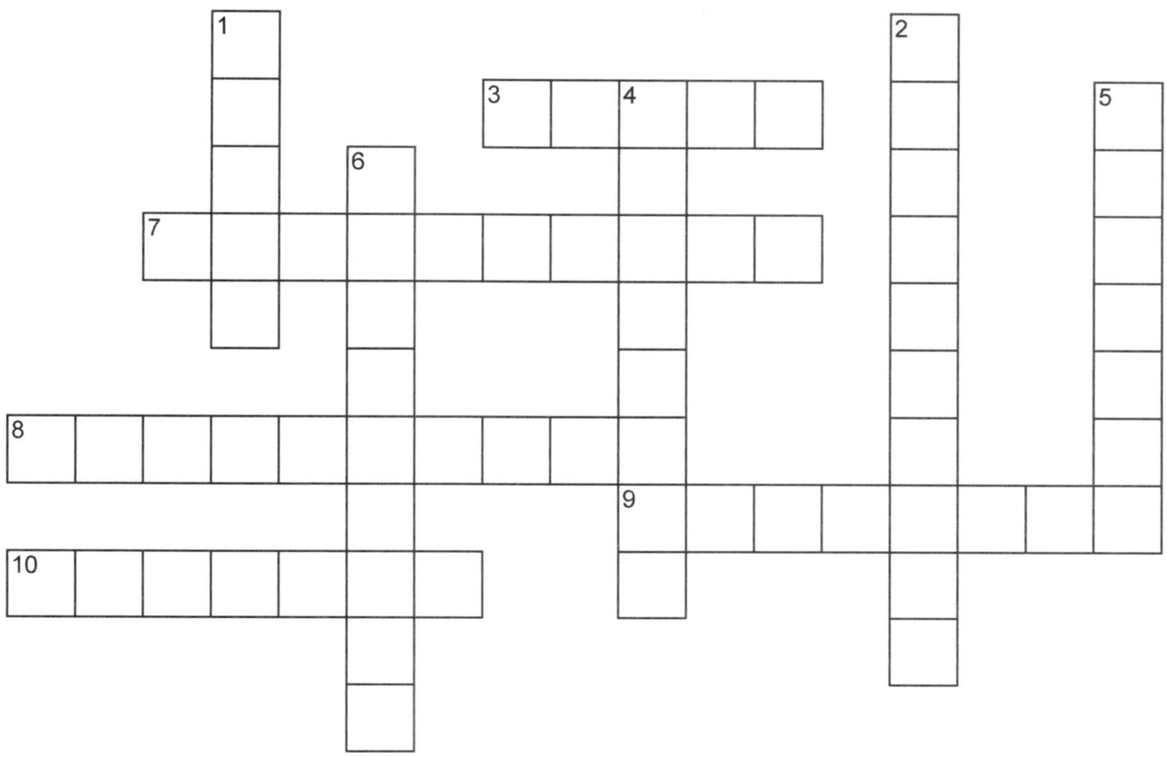

ACROSS

3 Yellow, clear, and amber plastic are types of these.

7 Dates for compounded preparations.

8 Important date in commercial product packaging.

9 Compounded preparation on a roller coaster.

10 Ingredient that could affect preparation stability.

DOWN

1 Semi-solid preparation package.

2 Normal expiration date for compounded preparations.

4 Used to wrap suppositories.

5 Help protect compounded preparation.

6 Should be light resistant, tightly sealed, and impervious to air.

Answers on page 43.

Exercise C – Short Answer Quiz

In the video/DVD, good and consistent record keeping was discussed as part of the documentation and labeling process.

A. The compounding notebook is one mechanism used by the pharmacy department to document how a preparation is compounded. Please list at least 10 of the 12 elements that need to be documented when preparing a compound.

B. The label information is guided by state and federal regulations. Please list all 11 elements that are required on a pharmaceutical label.

Answers on page 43.

Exercise D – Multiple Choice Questions

Select the best answer to each of the following questions.

1. **Ultraviolet light may cause all of the following with compounded preparations except**
   A. Degradation.
   B. Loss of potency.
   C. Enhanced potency.
   D. All of the above.

2. **Aluminum is good for wraps because it is**
   A. Soft and malleable.
   B. Inexpensive.
   C. Easy to use.
   D. All of the above.

3. **Ointment jars and tubes are designed to store all of the following except**
   A. Capsules.
   B. Gels.
   C. Creams.
   D. Pastes.

4. **Ointment jars and tubes are designed to protect ingredients from**
   A. Dark.
   B. Light.
   C. Sterility.
   D. Stability.

5. **Documentation of compounding is part of the pharmacy's**
   A. Question and answer session.
   B. Quality assurance program.
   C. Quality acuity program.
   D. All of the above.

6. **Labeling is part of which of the following?**
   A. Federal law.
   B. State law.
   C. Department policy.
   D. All of the above.

7. **Dates for compounded preparations should follow**
   A. USP/NF guidelines.
   B. ASHP guidelines.
   C. NABP guidelines.
   D. All of the above.

8. **Stability is defined as the extent to which a dosage form**
   A. Loses its original properties.
   B. Loses its contaminant properties.
   C. Retains its original properties.
   D. Retains its contaminant properties.

9. **All of the environmental factors listed below affect active ingredients, except**
   A. Light.
   B. Hydrogen.
   C. Temperature.
   D. Humidity.

10. **Storage requirements for compounded preparations must be in compliance with**
    A. The storage requirements of the active ingredient present in the largest amount.
    B. The storage requirements of the active ingredient present in the smallest amount.
    C. The storage requirements of the active ingredient with the strictest regulations.
    D. The storage requirements of the active ingredient with the most relaxed regulations.

Answers on page 43.

Exercise E – Fill in the Blank Exercises

1. Vials can protect contents from ______________ light.
2. Jars are usually filled using a ______________.
3. Tubes are usually filled using a ________________________.
4. The outside of containers or packages should be wiped with ______________ before labeling.
5. Compounded preparations must be ______________ and ______________ for patient use.
6. The __________________ is a list of ingredients and the procedure used in compounding the non-sterile preparation.
7. Proper ______________ of a compounded preparation coincides with labeling and is very important.
8. The ______________ of a preparation may change once ingredients are mixed together.
9. Drugs may become unstable due to mixing with another ingredient or improper ______________.
10. Expiration dates are determined by the stability of the drug and most are given in ______________.
11. Beyond-use dates are usually given in ______________ or ______________.
12. Proper storage ensures ______________ and ______________ of medications.
13. Follow ______________ guidelines when storing commercially available products.
14. Storage requirements help prevent ______________ and ______________ of all ingredients in medication.
15. Ingredients used in compounding should not be used beyond their __________________.

Answers on page 43.

Exercise F – Match Dosage Forms with the Correct Packaging

Match the compounded dosage form on the left with its package on the right.

_____ 1. Ointment	A. Aluminum wrap
_____ 2. Gel	B. Plastic bottle
_____ 3. Syrup	C. Amber vial
_____ 4. Capsule	D. Jar
_____ 5. Suppository	E. Glass bottle
_____ 6. Suspensions	F. Tube

Answers on page 43.

SECTION 4

Techniques

Learning Objectives

After watching the video/DVD, you should be able to

1. Recognize and define terminology related to compounding techniques.
2. Describe the various techniques demonstrated.
3. Identify when a certain technique would be used in compounding.
4. Discuss why the appropriate technique is important.
5. Match a compounded dosage form with its appropriate technique.
6. Discuss other elements to consider as part of the compounding process.

Exercise A – Word Search: Compounding Technique

Find the following words and circle them.

APOTHECARY
AVOIRDUPOIS
BACTERIA
CALIBRATION
CAPACITYRANGE
CAPSULESIZE
EUTECTICMIXTURES
GEOMETRICDILUTION
HANDWASHING
LEVIGATION
MEASURE
METRIC
MIXING
PROPERATTIRE
PUNCHMETHOD
SCRUBS
SOAPANDWATER
SPATULATION

L	N	G	F	T	Q	R	M	Q	V	V	Y	T	L	J	L	R	T	K	F	L
R	H	F	B	K	X	Y	E	Q	F	Y	J	K	T	Q	K	Z	M	P	F	Y
R	K	Z	N	L	V	J	W	T	H	V	N	T	R	X	F	C	L	T	K	Q
X	R	M	T	J	D	J	R	M	A	N	T	N	M	F	R	J	B	D	M	Y
R	L	I	M	N	L	L	R	K	O	W	P	Y	W	K	M	G	K	L	K	R
N	D	X	X	C	L	W	R	I	N	U	D	J	S	B	U	R	C	S	C	A
X	T	I	Q	K	X	B	T	F	N	V	W	N	M	M	G	D	R	W	A	C
F	L	N	N	D	D	A	N	C	N	M	C	K	A	E	D	B	C	N	P	E
F	H	G	Y	O	G	D	H	X	A	A	N	R	J	P	T	N	G	P	A	H
Y	T	L	R	I	I	M	H	J	P	L	N	M	W	L	A	R	P	T	C	T
N	B	V	V	W	E	T	B	S	V	F	I	M	H	F	P	O	I	P	I	O
T	R	E	T	T	W	L	U	Z	K	R	T	B	L	Z	Z	K	S	C	T	P
V	L	R	H	D	L	L	G	L	N	C	N	N	R	K	N	H	G	L	Y	A
L	T	O	M	M	E	N	J	L	I	O	L	J	T	A	V	L	N	D	R	G
Q	D	N	R	S	K	L	R	V	I	D	H	G	P	R	T	G	S	K	A	N
E	R	Z	I	M	N	K	B	T	K	F	C	V	P	M	N	I	M	K	N	I
R	H	Z	X	X	G	L	A	N	L	Y	M	I	Z	T	O	G	O	T	G	H
I	E	H	H	K	T	L	F	K	T	V	M	J	R	P	W	K	K	N	E	S
T	L	M	J	T	U	P	N	Q	R	P	M	R	U	T	R	X	R	C	V	A
T	B	G	F	T	F	Y	N	Y	Y	H	F	D	G	Z	E	K	J	N	F	W
A	X	N	A	N	R	N	R	P	G	C	R	B	V	T	M	M	N	P	J	D
R	C	P	P	N	K	T	B	F	N	I	F	R	L	B	W	K	O	F	Z	N
E	S	M	E	A	S	U	R	E	O	B	A	C	T	E	R	I	A	E	T	A
P	Z	Q	L	G	M	N	W	V	Z	Z	T	J	J	N	K	D	M	J	G	H
O	K	N	V	R	K	N	A	T	N	L	D	K	K	C	F	R	W	D	W	W
R	V	L	W	J	D	M	N	G	W	B	R	Q	F	Z	H	M	L	C	J	B
P	F	R	M	B	S	E	R	U	T	X	I	M	C	I	T	C	E	T	U	E

Answers on page 44.

Exercise B – Crossword Puzzle: Do You Know Your Compounding Techniques and Terminology?

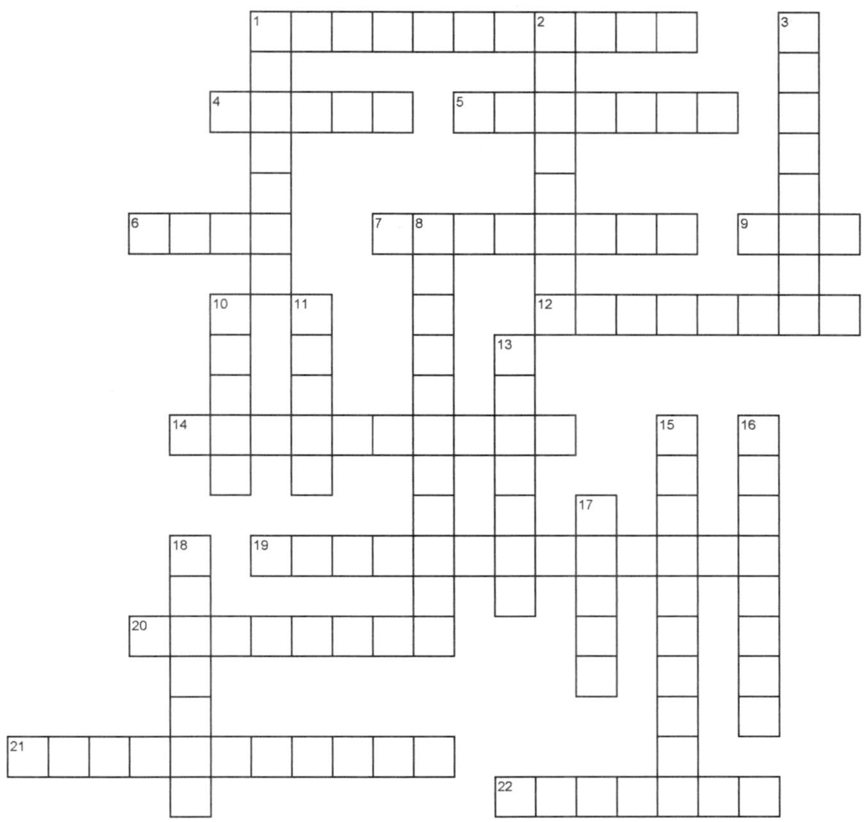

ACROSS

1 Method that does not reduce particle size.
4 Example of an emulsion.
5 Head, hand, face and foot coverings do this.
6 Material used to wrap lozenges, lollipops, and suppositories.
7 Can be found on all body surfaces.
9 Sensitivity of the class III balance in milligrams.
12 Method for mixing liquids.
14 Sorbitol and sodium bicarbonate are these kind of agents.
19 If shaped improperly these can cause patient discomfort.
20 Also known as trochees.
21 Should be weighed 100% accurately.
22 Lock this before adding or removing weight.

DOWN

1 Tool used during spatulation.
2 Another name for lozenges.
3 Produced when ingredients don't readily combine.
8 System strictly for weight measurement.
10 Product used as a suspending agent.
11 Suppositories should be uniform in size and this.
13 Pouring back and forth produces this kind of energy.
15 Process that utilizes a levigating agent.
16 Punch method is used to fill these.
17 Used to shape lollipops and medication sticks.
18 A calibrated measuring tool.

Answers on page 44.

Exercise C – Short Answer Quiz

In the video/DVD, proper hand washing was discussed and demonstrated. Because it is first and foremost when compounding, you should know the appropriate hand washing technique. Please list the steps in chronological order associated with proper hand washing technique.

1. ______________________________

2. ______________________________

3. ______________________________

4. ______________________________

5. ______________________________

6. ______________________________

Answers on page 44.

Exercise D – Multiple Choice Questions

Select the best answer to each of the following questions.

1. Types of measures used in compounding include
   A. Grams for weights.
   B. Liters for volume.
   C. Meters for length.
   D. All of the above.
2. The apothecary system of measurements includes all of the following, except
   A. Grains.
   B. Pints.
   C. Quarts.
   D. Ounces.
3. Percentage of errors when measuring are minimized by selecting the following:
   A. Largest container that will hold desired amount.
   B. Smallest container that will hold desired amount.
   C. Extra large container that will hold desired amount.
   D. Medium container that will hold desired amount.
4. Syringes are best for transferring what kind of liquid?
   A. Thin or oily.
   B. Thin or sticky.
   C. Thick or oily.
   D. Thick or sticky.
5. Which of the following devices are best for measurements when compounding?
   A. Household measuring devices.
   B. Workshop measuring devices.
   C. Calibrated devices.
   D. Non-calibrated devices.
6. The process by which particles are reduced to fine granules is known as
   A. Spatulation.
   B. Suspension.
   C. Geometric dilution.
   D. Trituration.
7. The process of mixing ingredients together with a spatula is known as
   A. Spatulation.
   B. Suspension.
   C. Geometric dilution.
   D. Trituration.
8. Trituration can be accomplished by which of the following?
   A. Crushing or pulverizing a single powder.
   B. Mixing equal amounts of more than one powder.
   C. Mixing unequal amounts of more than one powder.
   D. All of the above.
9. If an ointment slab is not available, then which of the following can serve as a substitute?
   A. Counter top.
   B. Parchment paper.
   C. Wax paper.
   D. Weighing paper.
10. Levigation is the process by which
    A. Water is added to powder one drop at a time to form a paste.
    B. Mineral oil is added to powder one drop at a time to form a paste.
    C. Powder is added to powder in small quantities at a time to form a paste.
    D. Cream is added to powder in small quantities at a time to form a paste.
11. Levigation is used when
    A. A dry ingredient must be introduced into a liquid base.
    B. A dry ingredient must be introduced into a dry base.
    C. A dry ingredient must be introduced into an ointment base.
    D. A dry ingredient must be introduced into an aromatic base.
12. Geometric dilution is the method used to
    A. Evenly triturate two or more ingredients that are unequal in quantity.
    B. Evenly triturate two or more ingredients that are equal in quantity.
    C. Reduce two or more ingredients to an unequal quantity.
    D. Reduce two or more ingredients to an equal quantity.
13. When performing the punch method, the powder should be
    A. ¼ to ½ the height of the empty capsule half.
    B. ½ to ¾ the height of the empty capsule half.
    C. ½ to full height of the empty capsule half.
    D. ¾ to full height of the empty capsule half.
14. When mixing liquids, it is best to pour
    A. The diluent into the active ingredient.
    B. The active ingredient into the diluent.
    C. The diluent into the filler ingredients.
    D. The active ingredient into the filler ingredients.
15. Suspensions are created when
    A. A granular medication is incorporated into an agent in which the medication turns into a liquid.
    B. A granular medication is incorporated into an agent in which the medication turns into a solid.
    C. A granular medication is incorporated into an agent in which the medication is soluble.
    D. A granular medication is incorporated into an agent in which the medication is insoluble.

Answers on page 44.

Exercise E – Fill in the Blank Exercises

1. Readability is the ____________ readable amount on a class III balance.
2. Capacity range is the ____________ readable amount on a class III balance.
3. The grain is the basic unit of measure for the ____________ system.
4. Patients should be provided with a calibrated ____________ or ____________ with which to measure their medication.
5. Always read the ____________ in order to measure liquids accurately.
6. Ingredients are usually spatulated on an ________________ .
7. Levigation may ____________ particle size because ingredients may also be triturated.
8. ______________ is the method by which a nonhomogenous mixture becomes a homogenous mixture.
9. Each capsule must be ____________ to ensure the correct amount is inside.
10. The smallest readable amount on a class III balance is _______________.
11. The largest readable amount on a class III balance is _______________.
12. An even and consistent mixture is called a ____________ mixture.
13. When choosing the correct capsule size, the ____________ size capable of holding the ingredients should be used.
14. Always prepare about __________ more worth of powder when compounding capsules.
15. The suspending agent used in a compounded preparation depends on the _______________.

Answers on page 44 and 45.

Exercise F – Match the Dosage Form with the Correct Technique or Preparation

Match the compounded dosage form on the left with the appropriate technique/preparation on the right.

_____ 1. Suspensions	A. Pouring/stirring
_____ 2. Capsules	B. Geometric dilution
_____ 3. Powders	C. Levigation
_____ 4. Pastes	D. Trituration
_____ 5. Creams	E. Spatulation
_____ 6. Liquids	F. Emulsion
_____ 7. Ointments	G. Punch method

Answers on page 45.

SECTION 5

Compounding Exercises

Pharmacy Compounding Log

Product Label

Pharmacy Lot Number

Date Prepared

Strength

Quantity Prepared

Quantity Packaged

Affix Pharmacy Label Here

	Manufacturer's Lot Number	Ingredient Name	Amount Needed	Measured By	Verified By
1					
2					
3					
4					
5					
6					
7					
8					

Directions for Preparation:

Completion Time: ____________________

Prepared By

Approved By

Date

Expiration Date

Auxiliary Labeling

Name: ______________________

300,000 Unit Nystatin Hard Lozenges

Materials: For Lozenge Base:

70g	Granular Sugar
40g	Light Corn Syrup
20mL	Distilled Water
to Taste	Flavoring
7 gtts	Food Coloring
1 Can	Cooking Spray
720mg	Nystatin Powder

1	Sauce Pan
1	Candy Thermometer
1	Hot Plate (heating up to 400 degree F)
1	Glass Stirring Rod
1	500ML Beaker
1	150mL Beaker
1	Lozenge Mold (10mL/lozenge)
	OR
12	Dose Cups with mL Demarcations
12	Individual Aluminum Wrappers

Prepares: 12 Lozenges

1. Prepare a hot water bath using tap water and a sauce pan.
2. Combine sugar, corn syrup, and water into 500mL beaker and place into the hot bath.
3. Constantly stir the solution until the sugar has melted and the temperature on the candy thermometer reads 300 degrees Fahrenheit (154 degrees Celsius).
4. Stir in desired color and flavoring.
5. Pour sugar solution into beaker, to a volume of 120mL.
6. Stir the solution and carefully add the nystatin powder, creating a homogeneous mixture.
7. Using the mold: lightly spray each lozenge slot with cooking spray, then fill each slot with 10mL of solution.
8. Using the cups: lightly spray each cup with cooking spray and fill each cup with 10mL of solution.
9. Allow lozenges to harden. (This may take several minutes.)
10. Remove lozenges from the mold or cup, wrap individually in aluminum.
11. Package, label, and prepare to dispense.

Estimated Time of Completion: 45 minutes

Name: ______________________

Zinc Oxide Paste

Materials:	25g	Zinc Oxide Powder
	25g	Cornstarch
	50g	White Petrolatum
	2mL	Mineral Oil (Levigating Agent)
	1	Mortar and Pestle
	1	Ointment Slab
	1	Class-A Balance and Counterweights
	1	Oral Syringe
	1	S/S Spatula

Prepares: 100g

1. Weigh ingredients.
2. Geometrically dilute zinc oxide using a mortar and pestle.
3. Levigate ZnO/cornstarch powder using mineral oil.
4. Spatulate the zinc oxide/cornstarch powder and white petrolatum into a paste.
5. Ensure a homogenous mixture by thorough spatulation.
6. Weigh and tare the empty ointment container.
7. Package the product to 30g.
8. Label and prepare product.

Estimated Time of Completion: 15 minutes

Name: ____________________

88% Isopropyl Alcohol

Materials:	16 fl.oz.	70% Isopropyl Alcohol, **OR**
	32 fl.oz.	Distilled Water
	16 fl.oz.	91% Isopropyl Alcohol
	1	Graduated Cylinders with sufficient capacity to measure required amounts of each ingredient
	2	500mL Beakers
	1	Medication Bottle with sufficient capacity to store requested quantity of product

Prepares: 360mL

1. Using alligation, calculate the amounts of 70% isopropyl alcohol or distilled water and 91% isopropyl alcohol needed to mix the preparation.
2. Using the graduate cylinder, measure the amount of 91% isopropyl alcohol needed and pour it into one beaker.
3. Using the graduate cylinder, measure the amount of 70% isopropyl alcohol, or distilled water, and pour it into the remaining empty beaker.
4. Pour the 91% isopropyl alcohol into the water, being careful not to splatter the liquid.
5. Pour the contents of the full beaker into the empty beaker.
6. Pour the liquids from one beaker to another several times to allow for a homogenous mixture.
7. Package, label, and prepare product for dispensing.

Estimated Time of Completion: 5 minutes

Name: ____________________________

Apple Pie Capsules

Materials:	1.5g	Ground Cinnamon
	4.6g	Sugar
	0.5g	Ground Nutmeg
	1.5g	Apple Pie Spice
	2g	Whole Cloves
	5	Size "00" Gelatin Capsules
	1	Mortar and Pestle
	1	Class-A Balance and Counterweights
	1	Ointment Slab
	1	Medication Bottle

Prepares: 5 450mg Capsules

1. Weigh ingredients.
2. Triturate cloves into a fine powder.
3. Geometrically dilute remaining ingredients with ground cloves.
4. Weigh and tare the capsule intended to be filled.
5. Using the "punch" method, fill the capsule to the requested weight.
6. Verify the weight of the capsule and add/remove contents as necessary until desired weight is reached.
7. Once correct, place the filled capsule into the medication bottle.
8. Repeat steps 4 through 7 for each capsule up to the requested quantity.
9. Label and prepare product for dispensing.

Estimated Time of Completion: 20 minutes

Name: ____________________

Metronidazole 500 mg/5 mL Oral Suspension

Materials:	35 to 40 tabs	Metronidazole 500mg
	QS	Syrpalta or other Available Syrup Agent
	1	Mortar and Pestle
	2 Sheets	Weighing Paper
	1	Class-A Balance with counter weights
	1	Medication Bottle with sufficient capacity to store requested quantity of product

Prepares: 160mL

1. Weigh 32 tablets of metronidazole 500mg and record this weight: ______________. *This is the amount of medication powder necessary to properly create a suspension at a concentration of 500mg/5mL in 160mL (160mL/5mL = 32).*
2. Triturate 35 to 40 tablets of metronidazole tablets.
3. Using the Class-A Balance, weight an amount of powder equal to the weight of 32 tablets as determined in step one.
4. Using weighting paper as a conical funnel into the medication bottle, carefully pour the triturated powder into the bottle.
5. Add a sufficient quantity of syrpalta or other pharmaceutical suspending agent to the desired volume of 160mL.
6. Shake well for at least 40 seconds.
7. Package, label, and prepare product for dispensing.

Estimated Time of Completion: 15 minutes

Name: ___________________________

Magic Mouthwash (4:2:1)

Materials:	4 parts	Diphenhydramine Syrup (12.5mg/5mL)
	2 parts	2% Lidocaine Viscous Jelly
	1 part	Mylanta, Unflavored or Mint Flavored
	3	Graduated Cylinders with sufficient capacity to measure required amounts of each ingredient
	1	Medication Bottle with sufficient capacity to store requested quantity of product

Prepares: QS

1. Calculate amount of each ingredient necessary to prepare the requested quantity.
2. Using one graduated cylinder per product, pour/measure the appropriate amount of each ingredient.
3. Add the ingredients to the medication bottle in the following order: 2% lidocaine, mylanta, diphenhydramine.
4. Seal the medication bottle and agitate the bottle as to homogeneously combine the ingredients (at least 40 seconds).
5. Label and prepare product for dispensing.

Estimated Time of Completion: 7 minutes

Answer Key

Section 1: **Dosage Forms**

Exercise A

P	K	S	E	R	U	T	C	N	I	T	Y	L	S	X	S	T	D
T	P	O	W	D	E	R	S	L	B	S	B	M	U	Y	N	P	E
N	N	S	M	R	W	M	Q	J	Y	K	R	C	S	V	O	K	M
L	D	K	U	Z	T	T	M	R	K	Y	F	E	P	B	I	P	U
R	N	Q	H	P	F	Y	U	C	F	J	X	C	E	P	T	S	L
N	Z	G	H	H	P	P	E	Z	L	T	T	V	N	H	U	T	S
X	W	N	L	N	S	O	W	L	R	L	C	F	S	B	L	N	I
V	H	K	M	L	J	W	S	A	I	M	V	E	I	L	O	E	O
C	R	E	A	M	S	Z	C	I	N	X	L	D	O	K	S	M	N
D	B	J	J	C	S	T	N	H	T	U	I	X	N	T	C	T	S
G	V	Z	Z	D	S	E	R	R	S	O	X	R	S	G	I	N	R
T	B	P	Q	N	R	C	G	P	P	H	R	E	S	K	T	I	C
T	Q	X	N	Z	R	T	A	N	L	K	T	I	Y	T	A	O	K
Z	V	T	J	V	C	C	Z	M	E	S	L	K	E	T	M	R	N
K	F	K	Y	L	M	L	Q	F	A	Z	P	B	M	S	O	X	G
B	L	P	D	D	T	H	B	P	M	R	O	N	M	F	R	W	R
J	S	N	O	I	T	O	L	M	L	C	M	L	X	T	A	N	J

Exercise B

Solution:

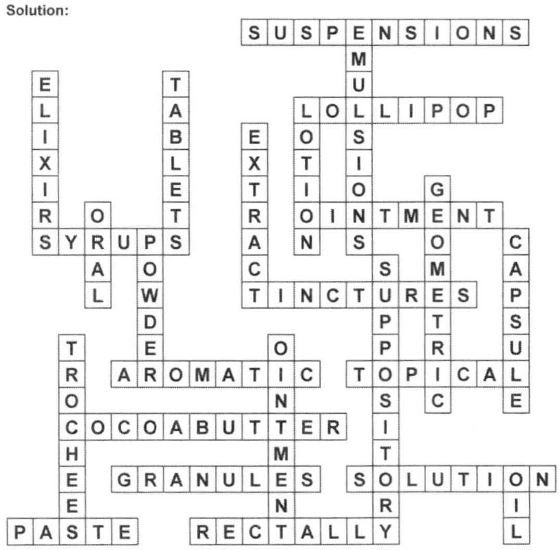

Exercise C

Make medications that are not commercially available.

Provide smaller doses for pediatric patients.

Add or mask flavors to make medications more appealing.

Provide veterinary medications.

Customize dosage forms for patients who cannot swallow.

Prepare specialized medications for specific diseases and conditions.

Exercise D

1. B
2. A
3. D
4. D
5. C
6. A
7. B
8. B
9. D
10. B
11. C
12. A
13. B
14. C
15. D

Exercise E

1. Active ingredient
2. Size, density
3. Melting, active ingredient
4. Undissolved
5. Tinctures
6. Hydroalcoholic
7. Syrups
8. Creams, lotions, ointments, and pastes
9. Water in oil
10. Aqueous
11. Alcohol
12. Shaken
13. Alcoholic, hydroalcoholic
14. Technique
15. Drug delivery system

Exercise F

1. C
2. D
3. E
4. A
5. B

Section 2: **Equipment**

Exercise A

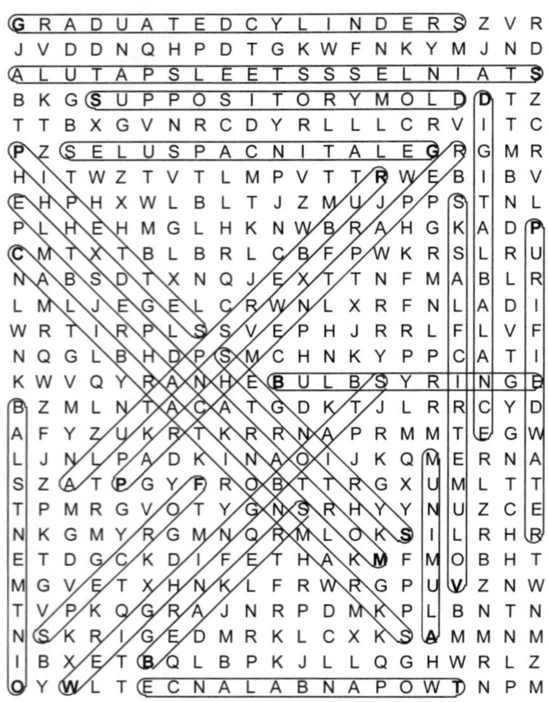

Exercise B

Solution:

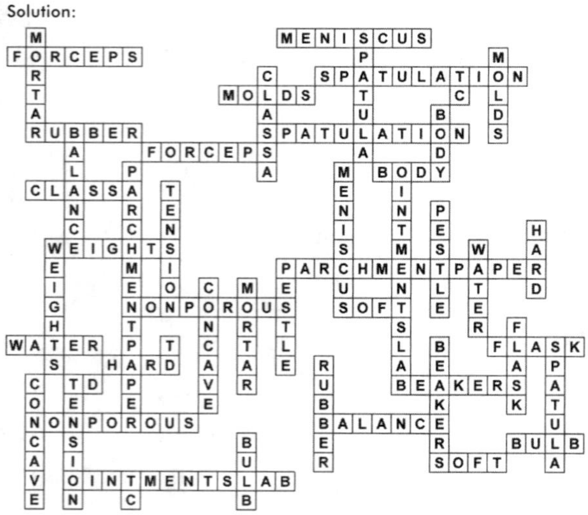

Exercise C

Suppository molds are necessary to provide the appropriate shape for the compounded suppository. The three most common types of molds are plastic, aluminum, and rubber.

Exercise D

1. A
2. D
3. B
4. C
5. D
6. B
7. A
8. D
9. A
10. A
11. D
12. B
13. C
14. C
15. B

Exercise E

1. Weighing papers
2. Digital balance
3. Graduated cylinders
4. Conical
5. Oral
6. Thicker
7. Punch
8. Rigid plastic
9. Transport
10. Ointment slab
11. Bowl, grinder
12. Wind cover
13. Fixed, partial
14. Deliver
15. Barrel, plunger

Exercise F

1. F
2. H
3. I

4. G
5. B
6. D
7. E
8. J
9. C
10. A

Section 3: **Packaging**

Exercise A

K	H	N	K	X	D	F	F	P	J	X	O	S	C	D
N	W	L	X	T	C	K	A	V	B	W	I	P	S	X
Y	Q	P	A	R	Z	C	D	L	R	R	N	A	E	Z
P	R	G	B	B	K	T	T	H	D	M	T	R	B	K
R	W	C	N	A	E	X	G	G	M	N	M	W	U	L
M	T	J	G	I	X	L	N	V	N	T	E	M	T	L
T	L	I	K	R	R	I	I	W	K	R	N	U	T	G
T	N	Q	H	L	T	O	W	N	L	W	T	N	N	L
G	R	X	N	A	Q	M	T	Q	G	T	J	I	E	V
X	J	T	D	T	M	K	L	S	N	T	A	M	M	X
L	D	Y	P	M	T	W	Q	Y	H	G	R	U	T	J
G	L	A	S	S	B	O	T	T	L	E	S	L	N	K
N	D	P	R	N	C	C	X	W	G	C	Z	A	I	L
L	N	N	O	I	T	A	T	N	E	M	U	C	O	D
S	E	L	T	T	O	B	C	I	T	S	A	L	P	N

Exercise B

Solution:

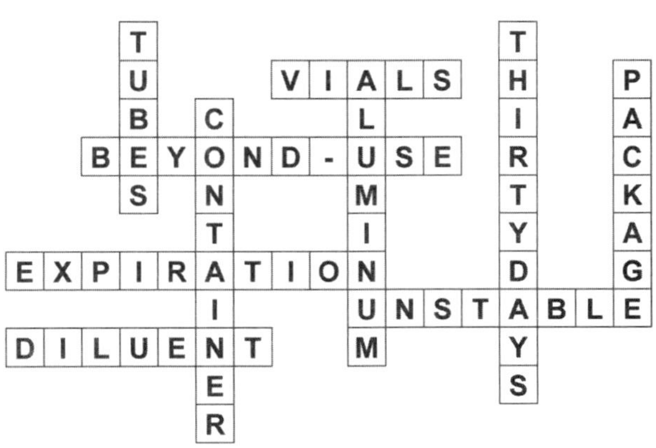

Exercise C

A. Label requirements, Formulas and procedures, Training, Equipment calibration, Equipment maintenance, Formulation record used, Date of preparation, Time of preparation, Beyond use date, Preparer's signature, Equipment used, and Quality control procedures used.

B. Pharmacy name, Pharmacy address, Pharmacy phone number, Prescription number, Patient name, Directions for use, Name of active ingredient, Quantity of active ingredient, Preparer's initials, Beyond use date, and Auxiliary labels.

Exercise D

1. C
2. D
3. A
4. B
5. B
6. D
7. A
8. C
9. B
10. C

Exercise E

1. Ultraviolet
2. Spatula
3. Filling bag
4. Alcohol
5. Safe, effective
6. Formulation record
7. Dating
8. Stability
9. Storage
10. Years
11. Days, months
12. Longevity, stability
13. Manufacturer's
14. Contamination, decomposition
15. Expiration date

Exercise F

1. D
2. F
3. E
4. C
5. A
6. B

Section 4: **Techniques**

Exercise A

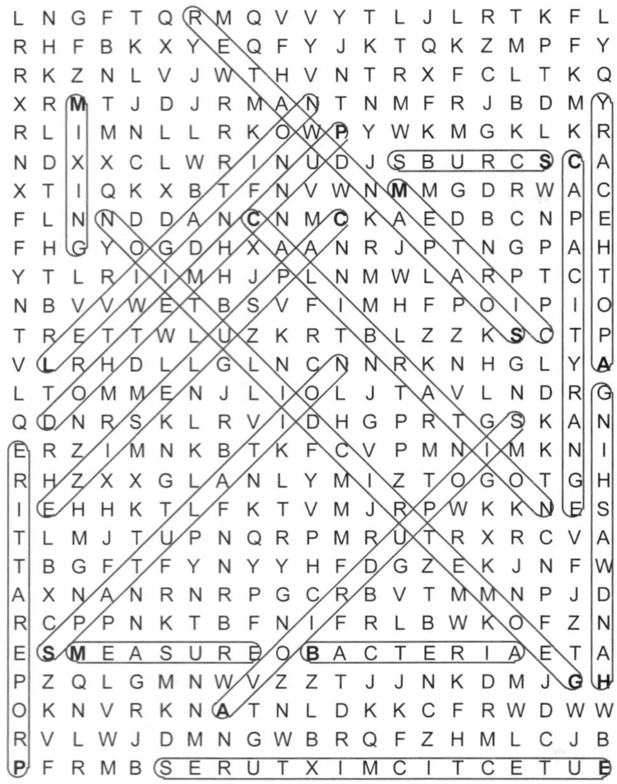

Exercise B

Solution:

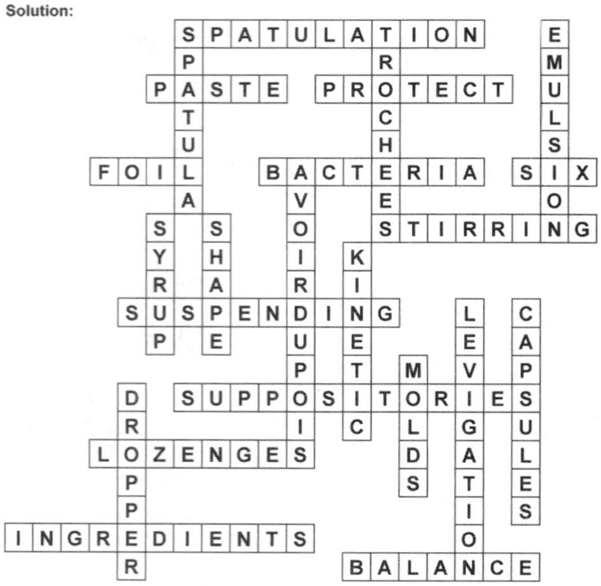

Exercise C

1. Remove all jewelry, including rings, bracelets, and watches.
2. Use warm water and let it run the entire time you are washing your hands.
3. Wet your hands and wrists up to your elbow.
4. Scrub hands, nails, wrists, and forearms thoroughly for at least 30 seconds with a brush, warm water, and appropriate bactericidal soap. Scrub your palms, backs of your hands, between your fingers (each one individually), under your nails, and around your cuticles.
5. Rinse your hands well, holding your hands upward toward the water so the dirty water and soap runs toward the elbows and not the hands. Hold fingernails under running water to make sure they are properly rinsed.
6. Use a clean lint-free towel to dry your hands and use the same towel to turn off the water. A touchless dryer system is preferred.

Exercise D

1. D
2. A
3. B
4. C
5. C
6. D
7. A
8. D
9. B
10. B
11. C
12. A
13. A
14. B
15. D

Exercise E

1. Smallest
2. Largest
3. Avoirdupois
4. Syringe, dropper
5. Meniscus
6. Ointment slab
7. Reduce

8. Geometric dilution
9. Weighed
10. 10 milligrams
11. 120 grams
12. Homogenous
13. Smallest
14. 10%
15. Active ingredient

Exercise F

1. D
2. G
3. B
4. C
5. F
6. A
7. E

Glossary

A

ACTIVE INGREDIENT
The chemical, substance, or other component of agents intended for use in the diagnosis, cure, mitigation, treatment, or prevention of diseases in humans or other animals or for use as nutritional supplements.

APOTHECARY
A system of weight that allows for fine weighing of medications such as aspirin, acetaminophen, and phenobarbital.

AROMATIC SOLUTION
A solution often with a sweet or pleasant aroma/smell.

ASHP
American Society of Health-System Pharmacists; a national professional association dedicated to representing, educating, and enhancing the profession and practitioners of pharmacy.

AUXILIARY LABEL
Used to give additional information. The required information on a prescription label does not provide sufficient information for every circumstance.

AVOIRDUPOIS
A system of weight in Great Britain and the United States, typically used for goods, medals, and medication. Units include the grain, ounce, and pound.

B

BACTERIA
A single-celled organism.

BEAKER
A cylindrical container with a pouring lip, used in a laboratory.

BEYOND-USE DATE
The maximum time period in which 90% or greater of a labeled active ingredient is measurable in the solution and container specified, under the stated storage or administration conditions.

BULB SYRINGE
A squeezable plastic ball-shaped device with an open tip, used in irrigation and to draw solutions into a laboratory device such as a pipette.

C

CALIBRATION
Adjusting a measuring instrument to make it accurate. The set of operations that establishes, under specified conditions, the relationship between values indicated by a measuring instrument or measuring system and the corresponding values of a quantity realized by a reference standard.

CAPSULES
Medication dosage form made of gelatin containing granules, powders.

CLASS A OR CLASS III BALANCE
A two-pan balance used to weigh small amounts of materials (often 120 g or less); these balances have a sensitivity of 6 mg.

COMPONENT
Any ingredient intended for use in the compounding of a drug preparation, including those that may not appear in such preparation.

COMPOUNDING
The preparation, mixing, assembling, packaging, and labeling of a drug or device in accordance with a licensed practitioner's prescription under an initiative based on the practitioner/patient/pharmacist/compounder relationship in the course of professional practice.

CONTAINER
That which holds the preparation and is or may be in direct contact with the preparation. The closure is part of the container.

CONTAMINATION
Any effect or action that has a negative impact on a preparation's integrity and makes it unfit for use.

CREAMS
A semi-solid dosage form used for topical application.

CROSS-CONTAMINATION
Transfer of microorganisms from one place to another.

D

DEMARCATION LINE
The boundary of a specific area.

DIGITAL BALANCE
A single-pan device used to weigh small amounts of materials.

DILUENT
A fluid or substance added to reconstitute or dissolve a substance.

DOCUMENTATION
A record of how a drug was processed and what quality attributes it possesses. (A written record of who did what and when.)

E

ELIXIRS
A sweet aromatic hydroalcoholic solution, used as a vehicle for pharmaceutical products.

EMULSIONS
A preparation containing two otherwise immiscible liquids.

EXPIRATION DATE
The date (and time, when applicable) beyond which the preparation should not be used (i.e., the preparation should be discarded beyond this date and time).

EXTEMPORANEOUS COMPOUNDING
The preparation of drugs or solutions that have no commercially available equivalents.

EXTRACTS
A solution containing the concentrated and active principles of a substance.

F

FORCEPS
A medical instrument used for holding objects.

G

GELATIN
Transparent, odorless, tasteless substance made from the boiling of ligaments, bones, and skin of animals, often porcine used for capsules.

GEOMETRIC DILUTION
Systematic process of combining two products using a mortar and pestle.

GRADUATED CYLINDER
A calibrated cylindrical device used in the measurement of liquid.

I

INCOMPATIBILITY
A physical or chemical phenomenon that reduces the concentration of the active ingredient(s).

INSTABILITY
The chemical processes that result in a degradation or change in the active ingredients.

L

LEVIGATION
The process of reducing solid particle size via the introduction of an emulsifying agent during the preparation of an ointment.

LOTIONS
A water-in-oil semi-solid dosage form containing insoluble or immiscible particles used in the application of topical products. Can be rubbed into the skin.

LOZENGES
A sweet-tasting solid dosage form absorbed through the lining in the mouth.

M

MORTAR
An instrument used in the mixing and grinding of pharmaceutical products; the bowl-shaped receptacle in a mortar and pestle set.

N

NABP
National Association of Boards of Pharmacy; a national association representing the Board of Pharmacy from each state in the United States.

O

OINTMENT
An oil-in-water semi-solid dosage form used in topically applied products that forms a barrier on the skin.

OINTMENT SLAB
A portable, reusable, square-shaped glass work surface on which pharmaceutical compounds are made; typically ¼ to 1¼ inches thick.

P

PARCHMENT PAPER
A portable, disposable, square shaped paper work surface on which pharmaceutical compounds are made.

PARTICULATES
Airborne particles found in the environment such as pollen, dust, bacteria, miscellaneous living and dead organisms, skin flakes, hair, clothing lining, cosmetics, respiratory gases, and bacteria from perspiration.

PASTES
A soft, smooth, and viscous starch-containing topical compound used in the preparation of pharmaceutical products.

PESTLE
An instrument used in the mixing and grinding of pharmaceutical products; the heavy tool used for grinding in a mortar and pestle set.

PIPETTE
A slender graduate tube used in the measurement and transfer of liquids in the laboratory.

POWDERS
A finely divided and triturated substance, from fine to coarse particles.

PROCEDURE
A "how to" document that provides methods for carrying out a policy. Procedures outline the complete cycle of a task, step by step, and assign responsibility to specific personnel.

PUNCH METHOD
A method used to fill gelatin capsules in pharmaceutical compounds. The body of the capsule is repeatedly punched into a cake of medication powder until full.

Q

QUALITY ASSURANCE GUIDELINES
Set of activities necessary to ensure that the processes used in the preparation of non-sterile drug preparations lead to preparations that meet predetermined standards of quality.

S

SPATULATION
A process by which ingredients are combined by spatulas, used in the preparation of semi-solid dosage forms.

STABILITY
The extent to which a preparation retains, within specified limits and throughout its period of storage and use, the same properties and characteristics that it possessed at the time of compounding.

SUPPOSITORY
A solid dosage form used in rectal, vaginal, or urethral administration of medication.

T

TINCTURES
An alcohol or alcohol-in-water based solution.

TRITURATION
The process of particle reduction when grinding substances with a mortar and pestle.

TROCHES
A small tablet or lozenge; see lozenge.

TWO-PAN BALANCE
See class-A or Class III balance.

U

USP/NF
United States Pharmacopoeia/National Formulary; a compendium of national standards for all prescription, over-the-counter, and dietary products as well as medical devices.

V

VIAL
A plastic or glass container with a rubber closure secured to its top by a metal ring.

W

WEIGHING BOAT
A soft, plastic vessel in which products may be stored or placed for use in the laboratory.

WEIGHING PAPER
A glassine sheet of paper in which products may be placed for use in the laboratory.

Index

A

ABBREVIATION
  "TO CONTAIN," 11
  "TO DELIVER," 11
ALUMINUM, 21
APOTHECARY MEASUREMENTS, 29
APPLE PIE CAPSULES, 38
AQUAPHOR, 6

B

BALANCE, 13, 14, 15
BEAKER, 13, 15
BENZOYL PEROXIDE, 5

C

CALAMINE, 7
CALIBRATED PIPETTES, 14
CAPACITY RANGE, 30
CAPSULE, 23, 30, 31, 38
COMPOUNDING, 5
  LOG, 34
  NOTEBOOK DOCUMENTATION, 20
COUGH SYRUPS, 6
CREAM, 3, 5, 7, 31
CROSSWORD PUZZLE
  DOSAGE FORMS, 3, 41
  EQUIPMENT, 11, 42
  PACKAGING, 19, 43
  TECHNIQUE, 27, 44
CYLINDRICAL GRADUATED CYLINDERS, 14

D

DIPHENHYDRAMINE SYRUP, 40
DOCUMENTATION, 20, 21
DOSAGE FORMS
  CROSSWORD PUZZLE, 3, 41
  FILL-IN-THE-BLANKS, 6, 41
  MATCHING, 7, 42
  MULTIPLE CHOICE, 5, 41
  QUIZ, 4, 41
  WORD SEARCH, 2, 41

E

EMULSION, 27
ENVIRONMENTAL FACTORS, 21
EQUIPMENT
  CROSSWORD PUZZLE, 11, 42
  FILL-IN-THE-BLANKS, 14, 42
  MATCHING, 15, 42–43
  MULTIPLE CHOICE, 13, 42
  QUIZ, 12, 42
  WORD SEARCH, 10, 42
EUCERIN, 6
EXPIRATION DATE, 19, 21, 22
EXTRACTS, 6

F

FILL-IN-THE-BLANKS
  DOSAGE FORMS, 6, 41
  EQUIPMENT, 14, 42
  PACKAGING, 22, 43
  TECHNIQUE, 30, 44–45

G

GEL, 23
GELATIN, 5
GEOMETRIC DILUTION, 6, 29
GLYCERIN, 7
GRADUATED CYLINDER, 13
GRAIN, 30

H–J

HAND WASHING, 28
HYDROCORTISONE, 7
ISOPROPYL ALCOHOL (88%), 37
JARS, 22

L

LABEL, 20, 21, 43
LEVIGATION, 27, 29, 30
LIDOCAINE JELLY, 40
LIQUIDS, 31
LOG, 34
LOTION, 3, 7
LOZENGES, 3, 5, 27, 35

M

MATCHING
DOSAGE FORMS, 7, 42
EQUIPMENT, 15, 42–43
PACKAGING, 23, 43
TECHNIQUE, 31, 45
MEASURES, 29
MEDICATION STICK, 3
MENISCUS, 11
METRONIDAZOLE ORAL SUSPENSION, 39
MOLDS, 12
MORTAR, 13, 14, 15
MOUTHWASH, 40
MULTIPLE CHOICE
DOSAGE FORMS, 5, 41
EQUIPMENT, 13, 42
PACKAGING, 21, 43
TECHNIQUE, 29, 44
MYLANTA, 40

N–O

NON-STERILE COMPOUNDING, REASONS FOR, 4, 41
NYSTATIN HARD LOZENGES, 35
OINTMENT, 5, 6, 7, 23, 31,
OINTMENT JARS/TUBES, 21
OINTMENT SLAB, 13, 15, 29
ORAL CAPSULE, 5
ORAL SUSPENSION, 39

P

PACKAGING
CROSSWORD PUZZLE, 19, 43
FILL-IN-THE-BLANKS, 22, 43
MATCHING, 23, 43
MULTIPLE CHOICE, 21, 43
QUIZ, 20, 43
WORD SEARCH, 18, 43
PARCHMENT PAPER, 14, 15
PASTE, 5, 6, 7, 31, 36
PESTLE, 13, 15
PETROLATUM, 36
PETROLEUM JELLY, 3, 36
PHENOBARBITAL ELIXIR, 5
PIPETTE, 13, 15
POWDERS, 5, 6, 31
PUNCH METHOD, 29

Q

QUIZ
- DOSAGE FORMS, 4, 41
- EQUIPMENT, 12, 42
- PACKAGING, 20, 43
- TECHNIQUE, 28, 44

R–S

READABILITY, 30
SCALE, 13
SLIP TIPS, 14
SODIUM BICARBONATE, 27
SORBITOL, 5, 27
SPATULA, 13, 15
SPATULATION, 27, 29
STABILITY, 21
STORAGE REQUIREMENTS, 21, 22
SUPPOSITORIES, 3, 5, 6, 7, 11, 19, 23, 27
SUPPOSITORY MOLD, 13
SUSPENDING AGENT, 27, 30
SUSPENSIONS, 6, 23, 29, 31
SYRINGE, 13, 14, 15, 29
SYRINGE TIP, 13
SYRPALTA, 39
SYRUP, 23

T

TECHNIQUE
- CROSSWORD PUZZLE 27, 44
- FILL-IN-THE-BLANK, 30, 44–45
- MATCHING, 31, 45
- MULTIPLE CHOICE, 29, 44
- QUIZ, 28, 44
- WORD SEARCH, 26, 44

THICKENING AGENTS, 6
TINCTURES, 6
TRIPLE ANTIBIOTIC, 7
TRITURATION, 29
TROCHEES, 27
TUBES, 22

U–V

ULTRAVIOLET LIGHT, 21
VASELINE, 6
VOLUMETRIC FLASK, 13

W–Z

WEIGHING BOATS, 14
WEIGHING PAPERS, 14, 15
WORD SEARCH
- DOSAGE FORMS, 2, 41
- EQUIPMENT, 10, 42
- PACKAGING, 18, 43
- TECHNIQUE, 26, 44

ZINC OXIDE, 7
ZINC OXIDE PASTE, 36